Don't Say I Didn't Tell You. Be Your Own Primary Care Physician (PCP)

Dr. Joseph Conteh

Table of Contents

Prologue

Don't Say I Didn't Tell You: Be Your Own PCP

Understanding that your health and wellbeing are your primary responsibilities is not just wisdom; it is an imperative for living a fulfilling and empowered life. A sound mind can only flourish in a sound body, and it is this synergy that forms the foundation of true wealth. No amount of financial success or material gain can replace the vitality and peace that come from being healthy and whole. The adage "health is wealth" is more than a cliché; it is a guiding principle that reminds us not to sacrifice our wellbeing in the relentless pursuit of external achievements. After all, wealth is meaningless without life, and life loses its quality without health.

Your Body, Your Responsibility

Your body is your most valuable asset, and understanding its needs, rhythms, and vulnerabilities is a task no one can perform better than you. While healthcare providers play an important role in diagnosing and treating illnesses, they rely on the information you provide. This makes you the primary architect of your health narrative. Regular self-care, diligent observation of your body, and a proactive approach to maintaining your wellbeing are indispensable. By investing time and effort in understanding and nurturing your body, you take the first steps toward preventing chronic conditions and avoiding the pitfalls of a healthcare system that sometimes prioritizes profits over patient care.

The Hidden Risks in Modern Healthcare

The U.S. healthcare system, despite its advanced technologies and skilled professionals, has a dark side that cannot be ignored. Medical errors have emerged as a significant issue, reportedly causing 251,000 deaths annually in the United States. That equates to 700 deaths a day—approximately 9.5% of all deaths. These errors, which range from medication mistakes to "never events" like operating on the wrong body part, highlight the fallibility of even the most trusted healthcare providers. Compounding this issue is the lack of mandatory reporting for deaths caused by medical errors, leaving many incidents unaccounted for. Patients are left vulnerable, often bearing the consequences of systemic flaws and individual negligence.

The Cost of Negligence

When medical professionals breach their duty of care, the consequences can be devastating. Patients harmed by such negligence or families who lose loved ones due to medical errors have the right to seek legal recourse. Medical malpractice lawsuits are a means to hold negligent parties accountable, but they are a reactive solution to problems that could often be avoided with proactive self-care and vigilance. The reliance on a system fraught with inefficiencies and errors underscores the importance of taking charge of your health.

Empower Yourself Through Awareness

The solution lies in shifting the paradigm of healthcare. Instead of being passive recipients of care, individuals must become active participants. This involves educating yourself about your health, seeking second opinions, and asking critical questions about prescribed treatments. Understanding your body's needs and investing in preventive care can significantly reduce your dependence on a flawed healthcare system. By becoming your own PCP, you minimize the risks associated with medical errors and ensure that decisions about your health align with your best interests.

A Call to Action

The insights shared here are not merely cautionary tales but a call to action. Your health is your greatest treasure, and safeguarding it requires effort, vigilance, and empowerment. While healthcare systems and professionals are valuable allies, the ultimate responsibility for your wellbeing rests with you. Commit to understanding, caring for, and treating your body with the respect it deserves. By doing so, you not only protect yourself from the pitfalls of profit-driven care but also take a stand for a life lived fully and healthily.

The book opens by challenging traditional notions of healthcare that place the primary responsibility for their healthcare in the hands of doctors and hospitals.

X

While professional medical care is essential, individuals play the most critical role in maintaining and improving their health. The central theme is empowerment: encouraging readers to take ownership of their well-being by becoming proactive participants in their healthcare journey.

Chapter 1: Understanding Your Body

Understanding your body is the cornerstone of proactive healthcare. It begins with the realization that your body constantly communicates with you, sending signals that reflect its state of well-being. These signals may be as subtle as changes in energy levels or as pronounced as persistent pain, yet many people overlook them or fail to interpret their significance. This chapter emphasizes the importance of developing a deeper awareness of these cues to maintain health and prevent potential illnesses.

The first step in understanding your body is recognizing its strengths and limitations. Everyone's physiology is unique, shaped by factors like genetics, lifestyle, and environment. By taking the time to observe and document how your body reacts to various situations—such as stress, diet, or exercise—you can begin to identify patterns. For instance, you may notice that certain foods make you feel lethargic or that consistent sleep deprivation triggers headaches. These observations form the foundation of self-awareness and help you make informed choices.

Another critical aspect of this chapter is learning to identify early warning signs of illness. Many serious health conditions, such as diabetes or hypertension, develop gradually, often without obvious symptoms. Paying attention to seemingly minor changes—like increased thirst, unexplained weight changes, or persistent fatigue—can alert you to underlying issues before they become more severe. Understanding these signals can empower you to seek medical advice early and take preventive actions.

Tracking personal health metrics is another valuable tool for self-awareness. Regularly monitoring factors like weight, blood pressure, heart rate, and glucose levels provides a tangible picture of your health. Advances in wearable technology and health apps have made it easier than ever to collect and analyze this data. By maintaining a record of these metrics, you can track changes over time and share valuable insights with your healthcare provider during check-ups.

Understanding your genetic predispositions is equally important. Your family history can offer clues about conditions you might be at risk for, such as heart disease, cancer, or autoimmune disorders. This knowledge allows you to take targeted preventive measures, like lifestyle modifications or early screenings, to reduce your risk. Genetic awareness is not about being fatalistic; it's about empowering yourself with information to make proactive decisions.

Listening to your body also involves tuning into your mental and emotional well-being. Stress, anxiety, and other psychological factors often manifest as physical symptoms, such as muscle tension, digestive issues, or difficulty sleeping. Recognizing the connection between your mental state and your physical health is key to maintaining balance and addressing issues holistically.

Developing self-awareness requires consistent effort and practice. One effective method is journaling your daily habits, feelings, and physical experiences. Over time, this habit can reveal patterns that you might otherwise miss. For example, you may notice that specific triggers, like certain foods or lack of exercise, coincide with recurring symptoms, such as bloating or fatigue.

The chapter also explores the concept of body literacy, which involves understanding how the body's systems interact. For example, knowing how the digestive system works can help you make better dietary choices, while understanding the cardiovascular system can inspire you to prioritize heart-healthy habits. Body literacy empowers you to approach your health with curiosity and confidence.

Self-awareness also extends to recognizing when something is out of the ordinary. While it's normal for the body to experience fluctuations, such as occasional aches or fatigue, persistent or unusual symptoms warrant attention. The chapter discusses the importance of trusting your instincts and seeking medical advice when you feel something isn't right, even if others dismiss your concerns.

The narrative highlights the importance of preventive care as a natural extension of self-awareness. When you understand your body's baseline, you are better equipped to make decisions that support long-term health. This includes everything from choosing nutrient-rich foods and engaging in regular exercise to scheduling routine health check-ups and screenings.

Understanding your body is not about obsessing over every detail but about cultivating a partnership with yourself. It's a process of learning to trust your observations, respect your limits, and celebrate your strengths. By developing this self-awareness, you lay the foundation for a healthier, more balanced life.

The chapter concludes by emphasizing that self-awareness is an ongoing journey. Your body is constantly changing, influenced by age, environment, and life circumstances. By remaining attentive and adaptable, you can continue to make informed decisions that support your well-being. In essence, understanding your body transforms you from a passive recipient of healthcare to an active participant in your health journey.

Listening to your body is an art that develops over time, and your experience illustrates how self-awareness can be a powerful tool in maintaining good health. Observing how your body reacts to food, drink, medication, and even environmental factors is an essential practice that not only fosters better health but also builds trust in your own instincts. Your ability to recognize patterns—like feeling weak and sick the day after consuming too much beer or noticing negative reactions to certain foods in specific locations—shows how closely tuning into your body's signals can guide you toward healthier choices.

This kind of self-awareness becomes a personal health map. By paying attention to how your body reacts, you learn to distinguish between what nourishes and supports you versus what disrupts your well-being. For example, you might notice that a particular meal leaves you feeling energized and alert, while another makes you lethargic and bloated. This simple yet profound act of observation allows you to make informed decisions that align with your unique needs, creating a personalized approach to health that no one else can replicate.

Many people have similar experiences with foods and drinks. Some find that consuming highly processed or sugary foods leads to a crash in energy levels, headaches, or even mood swings. Others might discover that specific types of alcohol, like beer or wine, cause them discomfort, while other beverages don't. Similarly, medications can vary widely in their effects depending on the individual.

Recognizing these patterns—perhaps a headache following a particular over-the-counter drug or an upset stomach after a new prescription—helps you take proactive steps, such as consulting your doctor about alternatives or adjusting your dosage under professional guidance.

Environmental factors also play a significant role in how we feel. Certain locations or climates can trigger allergies, fatigue, or other physical reactions. For instance, people often report feeling more tired or congested in areas with high pollution, while fresh mountain air might leave them invigorated. Some notice increased joint pain or stiffness in cold, damp weather, while others might feel unwell in high-altitude areas due to oxygen levels. Listening to these environmental signals and preparing accordingly—whether by adjusting diet, hydration, or clothing—demonstrates how in-tune you can become with your surroundings.

Your observation about alcohol is particularly relatable. Alcohol affects individuals differently depending on their metabolism, hydration levels, and even stress at the time of consumption. Drinking more than your body can handle often results in a "hangover," with symptoms like fatigue, nausea, and headaches. By recognizing your limits and understanding how alcohol impacts your body, you take the first step toward healthier habits, such as moderating consumption or avoiding triggers altogether.

These lessons extend beyond just food, drink, or location. For example, many people have noticed that engaging in certain activities—like sitting too long without breaks—can lead to back pain or stiffness. Similarly, neglecting hydration often results in sluggishness or headaches, while drinking enough water improves energy levels and focus. These simple observations are tools that help you make daily adjustments to support your health.

The beauty of listening to your body lies in the cumulative benefits. Over time, these small adjustments can have a profound impact on your overall health and well-being. For example, identifying that spicy foods cause acid reflux might lead you to avoid them, which in turn could improve your sleep quality and digestion. Similarly, understanding that high-sodium meals cause bloating and discomfort might inspire you to cook more meals at home, reducing your reliance on processed foods.

When you take this level of control over your health, you become your own best advocate. No healthcare provider, no matter how skilled, could feel what you feel or experience what you experience. They can offer guidance and expertise, but the day-to-day responsibility of making decisions about what to eat, drink, or avoid ultimately falls to you. By tuning into your body's unique responses, you become an informed and empowered participant in your own healthcare.

This process also allows for flexibility and adaptation. As your body changes over time—whether due to aging, lifestyle shifts, or new health challenges—your ability to observe and respond evolves as well. You might discover that foods or habits you tolerated well in your twenties no longer serve you in your forties. Staying in tune with these changes ensures that your self-care practices remain relevant and effective.

In conclusion, listening to your body and observing how it reacts to food, drink, medication, and environmental factors is the foundation of being your own primary care physician. It's about cultivating a partnership with your body, understanding its needs, and taking action to support its well-being. By combining these insights with professional medical advice when necessary, you create a comprehensive and personalized approach to health that empowers you to thrive. Your journey is a testament to the fact that no one knows your body better than you do, and this understanding is the ultimate key to long-term health and happiness.

The COVID-19 pandemic brought unprecedented challenges to global health, governance, and individual freedoms. While vaccines were developed and rolled out at remarkable speed, the process was not without controversy, especially concerning the rights of individuals to make informed decisions about their own bodies. Reports of adverse reactions, including deaths potentially linked to vaccines, fueled skepticism, and fear in many communities. These fears were particularly pronounced among individuals with preexisting health conditions, who worried about how the vaccine might interact with their unique medical profiles.

One significant point of contention during the pandemic was the perceived violation of human rights. Governments around the world implemented policies to encourage or mandate vaccination as a public health strategy to curb the virus's spread. While the intention was to protect public health, these measures sometimes overlooked individual autonomy. In many cases, people were faced with indirect coercion, where authorities and employers-imposed consequences for noncompliance. For example, employees in various sectors were threatened with termination or forced unpaid leave if they refused to get vaccinated, effectively depriving them of their livelihoods.

Educational institutions, too, became arenas for this debate. In several countries, universities mandated that students be vaccinated before attending in-person classes or accessing campus facilities. This created dilemmas for students who had concerns about the vaccine but feared losing their education or scholarships if they did not comply. Parents faced similar challenges when schools required vaccination for children to continue attending, placing families in difficult positions regarding their health decisions and children's education.

Travel restrictions were another area where individual rights were compromised. Many governments introduced vaccine passports as prerequisites for international travel, barring unvaccinated individuals from crossing borders or attending events. While intended to ensure safer interactions, these policies raised ethical concerns about freedom of movement and access to global opportunities. Those unable to take the vaccine for medical reasons or personal beliefs were effectively excluded from participating in significant aspects of life.

The situation was even more dire in certain industries, such as healthcare, where vaccination mandates were strictly enforced. Frontline workers, who had risked their lives during the early phases of the pandemic, were faced with ultimatums: get vaccinated or lose their jobs. This not only demoralized many workers but also created staffing shortages in critical sectors, exacerbating an already strained healthcare system.

In some countries, the push for vaccination extended to public benefits. Governments threatened to withhold social services, welfare payments, or unemployment benefits from unvaccinated individuals. Such policies disproportionately affected vulnerable populations who relied on these benefits for survival, leaving them with little choice but to comply, even if they had legitimate concerns about their health.

Religious and cultural beliefs also became battlegrounds for vaccine mandates. Some individuals objected to vaccination on the grounds of deeply held convictions, yet they found their beliefs dismissed or disregarded by authorities. In certain cases, exemptions for religious or personal beliefs were denied outright, forcing individuals to choose between their faith and compliance with government regulations.

These policies led to widespread protests and legal battles in many countries. Individuals and advocacy groups argued that such mandates violated constitutional rights, including freedom of choice, bodily autonomy, and the right to work. Courts in various jurisdictions issued mixed rulings, with some upholding vaccine mandates as necessary for public health and others striking them down as unconstitutional.

The issue of vaccine equity further complicated the narrative. In low-income countries, where vaccine access was limited, people who wanted to be vaccinated could not get the shots, highlighting a stark disparity. Meanwhile, in wealthier nations, individuals who refused vaccination were criticized, creating divisions and stigmatization within societies. This disparity underscored the uneven burden of the pandemic and raised ethical questions about how health policies were applied globally.

As the pandemic progressed, the debate over vaccine mandates evolved into a broader discussion about the balance between public health and individual rights. While the vaccines undoubtedly saved countless lives and reduced the severity of COVID-19 in many cases, the methods used to enforce vaccination policies left lasting scars on societal trust. Governments, employers, and institutions were seen as overstepping boundaries, prioritizing collective goals over personal freedoms in ways that many found unacceptable.

In reflecting on these experiences, it becomes clear that public health strategies must balance efficacy with respect for individual autonomy.

Education and transparency about vaccine safety, coupled with accommodations for medical, cultural, and personal concerns, can foster trust and collaboration rather than coercion. The pandemic highlighted the importance of listening to people's fears and ensuring that public health policies are inclusive, respectful, and equitable, especially during times of crisis.

During the COVID-19 pandemic, many individuals around the world turned to home remedies as a means of prevention and self-care. Faced with limited access to healthcare facilities, overwhelmed hospitals, and the uncertainty surrounding the virus, people sought natural and readily available solutions to support their immune systems and protect their health. These self-care practices often reflected a deep understanding of the body's needs and demonstrated the resilience of communities in times of crisis.

From herbal teas to dietary changes, home remedies varied widely across cultures and regions, often rooted in traditional medicine and ancestral knowledge. In parts of Asia, for instance, people turned to turmeric, ginger, and honey mixtures for their anti-inflammatory and immune-boosting properties. Similarly, in Africa, concoctions of neem leaves, moringa, and garlic were widely consumed, believed to combat viral infections and improve overall health. These remedies were passed down through generations, and during the pandemic, they gained renewed relevance.

In many households, vitamin-rich foods became staples. Citrus fruits, known for their high vitamin C content, were widely consumed to strengthen immunity. Other dietary shifts included increasing the intake of zinc-rich foods like seeds and nuts and incorporating anti-viral ingredients like oregano and thyme into meals. These adjustments not only addressed immediate health concerns but also improved long-term nutrition for many individuals.

Steam inhalation and saltwater gargling became common practices in numerous regions. People believed that steam inhalation, often infused with essential oils or herbs like eucalyptus, could help clear the respiratory tract and reduce viral load. Saltwater gargling, a traditional remedy for sore throats, was widely adopted to prevent infections in the throat and upper respiratory system. These methods, while simple, brought a sense of control and agency to people grappling with an unpredictable virus.

In South Asia, the ancient practice of "kadha," an herbal decoction made with ingredients like basil, clove, cinnamon, and black pepper, gained popularity. These drinks were consumed to enhance immunity and address respiratory symptoms. Ayurveda practitioners recommended daily routines for boosting immunity, including oil pulling, yoga, and breathing exercises, all of which became part of many people's self-care regimens.

Traditional remedies were complemented by modern approaches to self-care, such as staying hydrated, ensuring adequate rest, and reducing stress. Recognizing the impact of mental health on physical well-being, many people turned to meditation, mindfulness practices, and prayer to cope with the fear and uncertainty of the pandemic. These practices reinforced the idea that health is holistic, encompassing both the body and the mind.

The effectiveness of these home remedies was widely debated, but many individuals attributed their survival and well-being to these practices. Anecdotal reports of people recovering or avoiding severe symptoms after relying on traditional remedies spread quickly, creating a sense of hope and solidarity. In regions where healthcare systems were overwhelmed, such practices were not just a choice but a necessity.

At the same time, reports of deaths in hospitals during the pandemic heightened people's fears of institutional healthcare. Overcrowding, lack of resources, and limited medical knowledge about COVID-19 in its early stages contributed to high mortality rates in healthcare facilities. This stark reality further fueled the reliance on home remedies, as many individuals sought to avoid hospitalization at all costs.

The pandemic also revealed the ingenuity of people in adapting and sharing knowledge. Social media platforms became hubs for exchanging tips on natural remedies and self-care practices. Communities came together to share recipes, advice, and stories of resilience, demonstrating the power of collective wisdom in navigating a global health crisis.

However, this shift toward self-cure also underscored disparities in healthcare access and systemic shortcomings. While home remedies provided a sense of empowerment, they were not a substitute for comprehensive healthcare. Many individuals who relied solely on these remedies faced challenges when symptoms worsened and required professional medical attention. The lack of proper medical guidance sometimes led to delayed treatment and, in some cases, preventable deaths.

The experience of the pandemic highlighted the importance of a balanced approach to health. While self-care and home remedies played a crucial role in supporting immunity and managing mild symptoms, they also underscored the need for accessible and reliable healthcare systems. Governments and health organizations could learn from this experience by integrating traditional knowledge into public health strategies, providing clear guidelines for the safe use of home remedies, and addressing the gaps in healthcare access.

In retrospect, the widespread adoption of home remedies during COVID-19 reflects the resilience and resourcefulness of people in the face of adversity. It also serves as a reminder of the importance of understanding one's body and taking proactive steps to maintain health. While the pandemic challenged healthcare systems globally, it also reinforced the value of self-awareness, natural remedies, and the collective strength of communities in safeguarding their well-being.

Chapter 2: The Pillars of Preventative Care

Preventative care is the foundation of a healthy and fulfilling life, emphasizing proactive measures to maintain well-being and avoid chronic illnesses. This chapter introduces readers to the five core pillars of health: nutrition, exercise, sleep, stress management, and hydration. These interconnected elements form the backbone of a lifestyle that supports longevity and vitality, demonstrating how small, consistent changes can yield significant benefits over time.

Nutrition serves as the first and perhaps most critical pillar. What we consume fuels every cell in our body, influencing energy levels, immunity, and even mental clarity. A balanced diet rich in whole foods, such as fruits, vegetables, whole grains, lean proteins, and healthy fats, lays the groundwork for optimal health. The chapter explores how specific nutrients contribute to bodily functions—calcium for strong bones, fiber for digestive health, and antioxidants for combating inflammation. Readers are encouraged to adopt sustainable eating habits, such as planning balanced meals, reducing processed foods, and eating mindfully to better understand their body's hunger and fullness cues.

Exercise is the second pillar, vital for maintaining a strong and resilient body. Regular physical activity strengthens the heart, improves circulation, and supports mental well-being by reducing stress and boosting mood. This chapter provides guidance on incorporating exercise into daily life, no matter the fitness level or schedule. From brisk walking to strength training, readers are shown how achievable fitness goals can lead to transformative results. Emphasis is placed on finding enjoyable activities, whether it's dancing, swimming, or gardening, to ensure consistency and long-term commitment.

The third pillar, sleep, is often underestimated despite its profound impact on overall health. Quality sleep is when the body repairs itself, consolidates memories, and restores energy. The chapter delves into how poor sleep habits can lead to a weakened immune system, increased risk of heart disease, and impaired cognitive function. Readers are guided on how to establish a bedtime routine, optimize their sleeping environment, and address common issues like insomnia. Practices such as limiting screen time before bed and maintaining consistent sleep schedules are highlighted as effective strategies for improving rest.

Stress management is the fourth pillar, addressing the often-overlooked relationship between mental and physical health. Chronic stress can lead to a host of health issues, including high blood pressure, digestive problems, and depression. This chapter underscores the importance of recognizing stress triggers and developing coping mechanisms. Techniques like mindfulness meditation, deep breathing exercises, and engaging in hobbies are introduced as practical ways to reduce stress. Readers are reminded that while stress is an inevitable part of life, how they respond to it determines its impact on their health.

Hydration, the fifth pillar, is a simple yet crucial component of preventative care. Water is essential for every bodily function, from regulating temperature to flushing out toxins. Dehydration, even mild, can lead to fatigue, headaches, and poor concentration. The chapter explains the importance of drinking adequate water daily and provides tips for making hydration a habit, such as carrying a reusable water bottle and incorporating hydrating foods like cucumbers and oranges into meals. The benefits of proper hydration, including improved skin health, enhanced digestion, and increased energy, are highlighted to motivate readers.

Throughout the chapter, the interconnectedness of these pillars is emphasized. For example, how poor sleep can lead to overeating or how regular exercise can improve stress management and sleep quality. By understanding how these elements work together, readers are empowered to make informed decisions about their health. They are shown that preventative care is not about perfection but about progress—taking small steps each day to support their well-being.

Practical advice is woven throughout the narrative to help readers implement these pillars into their lives. Tips for creating meal plans, setting realistic fitness goals, and building a relaxing bedtime routine are presented in a relatable manner. The chapter acknowledges that life's demands can make health a low priority, but it encourages readers to view self-care as an investment in their future. Making even minor adjustments—like adding an extra serving of vegetables to meals or setting aside 10 minutes for stretching—can have profound long-term effects.

The chapter concludes by reinforcing the importance of consistency. Readers are reminded that health is a journey, not a destination, and that the pillars of preventative care are tools for navigating this journey. By committing to small, sustainable changes, individuals can take control of their health and significantly reduce the risk of chronic diseases. The chapter sets the stage for a deeper exploration of each pillar in subsequent sections, laying the foundation for a comprehensive approach to well-being.

Chapter 3: Building Your Personal Health Toolbox

Taking charge of your health requires not only knowledge but also the right tools and resources to support informed decision-making. A personal health toolbox is a collection of practices, technologies, and strategies that empower individuals to monitor, manage, and improve their well-being. This chapter explores how everyone can create and customize their health toolbox, equipping themselves with practical solutions that align with their needs and goals.

Keeping health records is a foundational element of this toolbox. Accurate and up-to-date records of personal and family medical histories provide invaluable insights that can guide healthcare decisions. By tracking past diagnoses, medications, allergies, and vaccinations, individuals can ensure that medical professionals have a clear picture of their health status during consultations. For example, knowing a family history of diabetes or heart disease can encourage earlier screenings and lifestyle adjustments. This chapter provides strategies for organizing health records, whether through traditional paper filing systems or digital platforms, and highlights the importance of sharing these records with trusted healthcare providers.

Monitoring devices are another vital component of the personal health toolbox. Advances in technology have made it easier than ever to track key health metrics from the comfort of home. Devices such as blood pressure monitors, glucometers, and pulse oximeters allow individuals to monitor their health regularly and detect early signs of potential issues. For instance, someone with hypertension can use a blood pressure monitor to track daily readings and identify patterns, which can help guide dietary or medication adjustments. Similarly, diabetics can benefit from glucometers to maintain steady glucose levels. This chapter explains how to use these devices effectively, interpret the data they provide, and integrate them into daily routines.

Fitness trackers and wearable technology add another layer of utility to health management. These devices track steps, heart rate, sleep patterns, and even stress levels, offering a comprehensive view of overall well-being. The chapter discusses how fitness trackers can motivate individuals to meet daily activity goals and foster a sense of accountability. Whether it's a beginner aiming for a 10,000-step goal or an athlete monitoring recovery time, these tools cater to a wide range of health and fitness objectives.

Health apps and technology further expand the capabilities of a personal health toolbox. With the explosion of mobile apps designed for health and wellness, individuals can now access a variety of tools to track diet, exercise, medication adherence, and mental health. For example, calorie-tracking apps help users make smarter dietary choices, while guided meditation apps promote mindfulness and stress reduction. This chapter reviews some of the most user-friendly and effective apps available, providing readers with options tailored to their needs. Additionally, it highlights apps that sync with wearable devices, creating an integrated health monitoring ecosystem.

Beyond tracking and monitoring, the chapter emphasizes the importance of scheduling and reminders as part of the health toolbox. Many apps and devices include features that send notifications for taking medication, scheduling doctor's appointments, or completing daily hydration goals. These reminders help individuals stay consistent with their health routines, reducing the likelihood of missed treatments or neglected self-care practices.

A well-rounded health toolbox also includes access to reliable health information. The chapter advises readers on how to evaluate online resources for credibility, distinguishing evidence-based medical advice from misinformation. It encourages individuals to consult reputable websites, such as those run by government health departments or academic institutions, and to stay updated on advancements in healthcare relevant to their conditions or goals.

Telemedicine has also emerged as a powerful tool in personal health management, particularly in the wake of the COVID-19 pandemic. The chapter discusses how virtual consultations with healthcare providers have made access to care more convenient and accessible, especially for routine check-ups or follow-ups. It provides tips for preparing for telemedicine appointments, such as having health records and questions ready, to make the most of the time with the provider.

The chapter also emphasizes customization and adaptability when building a personal health toolbox. Not all tools work for everyone, and individuals should experiment with different devices, apps, and practices to find what suits them best. A toolbox should evolve over time, incorporating new technologies or strategies as needs change. For instance, someone managing a temporary condition might rely on a specific app or device that becomes less relevant once they recover, allowing them to shift focus to other aspects of health.

Throughout the chapter, the theme of empowerment resonates strongly. By equipping themselves with these tools, individuals take an active role in their health journey, fostering a sense of control and confidence. The toolbox is not just about convenience; it's about creating a proactive approach to health that complements professional medical care.

The chapter concludes with practical advice on getting started. Readers are encouraged to identify their health priorities—be it weight management, chronic condition monitoring, or stress reduction—and select tools that align with those goals. By assembling and maintaining a personal health toolbox, individuals are better prepared to navigate the complexities of modern healthcare, achieve their wellness objectives, and lead healthier, more informed lives.

Chapter 4: Nutrition as Medicine

Nutrition lies at the heart of health and well-being. What we eat has a profound impact on our bodies, influencing everything from energy levels and immunity to the prevention and management of chronic diseases. In this chapter, we explore how food can be more than sustenance—it can be a powerful tool for healing, prevention, and vitality. By understanding the role of nutrition and making informed dietary choices, individuals can harness the power of food as medicine to improve their lives.

The Role of Nutrition in Preventing Chronic Diseases

The connection between nutrition and chronic illnesses like obesity, diabetes, and heart disease is undeniable. Diets high in processed foods, sugars, and unhealthy fats contribute to these conditions, while nutrient-rich whole foods help mitigate them. For example, fiber-rich foods such as oats, legumes, and vegetables can lower cholesterol levels and reduce the risk of heart disease. Similarly, lean proteins and low-glycemic carbohydrates are essential for managing blood sugar levels in diabetics. This section delves into how different foods impact the body and explains why making the right dietary choices is a critical step in preventing disease.

Understanding Macronutrients: The Building Blocks of Health

Macronutrients—proteins, carbohydrates, and fats—are the foundation of any diet, and understanding their roles can help individuals make balanced meal choices. Proteins, found in foods like chicken, beans, and fish, are crucial for tissue repair and muscle growth. Carbohydrates, particularly those from whole grains and vegetables, provide energy, while healthy fats from sources like avocados, nuts, and olive oil support brain function and hormonal balance. This section explains the optimal distribution of macronutrients for various health goals and lifestyles, emphasizing the importance of quality over quantity in dietary choices.

The Power of Micronutrients and Superfoods

Micronutrients—vitamins and minerals—play a vital role in maintaining optimal health. Calcium and vitamin D strengthen bones, magnesium supports nerve function, and antioxidants like vitamin C combat inflammation. Superfoods, which are nutrient-dense foods with exceptional health benefits, take center stage in this section. Blueberries, for instance, are packed with antioxidants that protect against cellular damage, while spinach provides iron and folate essential for blood health. Practical tips for incorporating superfoods into daily meals, such as blending leafy greens into smoothies or sprinkling flaxseeds onto yogurt, make it easy for readers to enhance their diets.

Reading Food Labels: Decoding What You Eat

Navigating modern food packaging can be overwhelming, with labels full of numbers, percentages, and hard-to-pronounce ingredients. This section teaches readers how to interpret food labels to make informed choices. It explains serving sizes, calorie counts, and the breakdown of macronutrients. The chapter also highlights red flags, such as high sugar content or artificial additives, that can undermine health goals. With this knowledge, readers can confidently select foods that align with their nutritional needs and avoid misleading marketing claims.

Nutrition for Disease Management

Food plays a therapeutic role in managing existing health conditions. For individuals with diabetes, focusing on low-glycemic foods like quinoa and lentils can help stabilize blood sugar levels. For those with hypertension, a diet rich in potassium-packed foods like bananas and sweet potatoes can help regulate blood pressure. Heart disease patients benefit from omega-3 fatty acids found in salmon and walnuts, which support cardiovascular health.

This section provides tailored dietary recommendations for managing common conditions, empowering readers to use nutrition as a complement to medical treatments.

Practical Tips for Healthy Eating

Making healthier dietary choices doesn't require drastic changes; small, consistent steps can have a significant impact. This section offers guidance on meal planning, such as incorporating more whole foods into each meal and gradually reducing processed items. Simple strategies like prepping ingredients in advance or using portion control can make healthy eating more accessible. Readers are encouraged to experiment with new recipes and cuisines to keep their diet varied and enjoyable.

The Importance of Hydration in Nutrition

Hydration is often overlooked in discussions about nutrition, yet it is equally vital for overall health. Water aids digestion, regulates body temperature, and supports cellular function. This section discusses how staying hydrated complements a nutritious diet and offers practical advice on meeting daily hydration needs. For those who find plain water unappealing, infused water with fruits like lemon or cucumber is suggested as an alternative.

Addressing Common Myths and Misconceptions

The world of nutrition is rife with myths and conflicting advice, which can confuse and mislead individuals. This section addresses common misconceptions, such as the fear of fats or the idea that carbohydrates should be completely avoided. By presenting evidence-based information, readers are guided toward balanced, sustainable approaches to nutrition that align with their health goals.

The Emotional and Social Aspects of Food

Food is not just fuel for the body; it is deeply tied to emotions, culture, and social connections. This section explores how to maintain a healthy relationship with food, free from guilt or restrictive dieting. It discusses the importance of mindful eating, savoring meals, and respecting cultural traditions while making health-conscious choices. Readers are encouraged to view food as a source of joy and nourishment rather than a source of stress.

The Lifelong Benefits of Nutritional Awareness

The chapter concludes by emphasizing that nutrition is a journey, not a destination. By understanding and prioritizing nutrition, individuals can prevent illness, manage chronic conditions, and improve their quality of life. Readers are reminded that small changes made today can lead to significant benefits over time, laying the foundation for a healthier future.

This chapter empowers readers to see food as medicine—a tool that can heal, energize, and transform. With the knowledge and practical advice provided, they are equipped to take control of their diets and, in turn, their overall health.

Chapter 5: Movement Is Medicine

Physical activity is one of the most powerful tools for maintaining health and preventing disease. Movement does more than just burn calories; it strengthens the body, sharpens the mind, and promotes emotional well-being. This chapter explores the profound impact of regular exercise on overall health and provides readers with practical guidance on how to make movement a natural and enjoyable part of their daily lives.

The Science Behind Exercise and Health

Exercise is not just about weight management—it is a cornerstone of disease prevention and physical resilience. Scientific research consistently shows that regular physical activity reduces the risk of chronic conditions such as hypertension, arthritis, heart disease, and diabetes. It improves circulation, strengthens muscles and bones, and enhances flexibility, making daily tasks easier and reducing the likelihood of injury. The chapter explains how movement positively impacts bodily systems, such as improving cardiovascular function, reducing inflammation, and enhancing the efficiency of metabolism.

Movement as a Preventative Measure

The role of exercise in preventing diseases like hypertension and arthritis cannot be overstated. Physical activity helps regulate blood pressure by improving the elasticity of blood vessels and promoting heart health. For those prone to arthritis, movement keeps joints lubricated, reduces stiffness, and strengthens the muscles that support joints. Even moderate activity, such as walking or gardening, can have a profound effect on reducing the risk of these conditions. Readers are encouraged to view exercise not as a luxury but as a critical component of preventative care.

The Emotional Benefits of Movement

Exercise is as much about mental health as it is about physical well-being. Engaging in regular activity releases endorphins, the body's natural "feel-good" chemicals, which elevate mood and reduce stress. Exercise has been shown to alleviate symptoms of anxiety and depression, providing a natural and effective way to improve emotional resilience. This section explores how movement creates a sense of accomplishment, builds confidence, and fosters emotional balance, turning exercise into a powerful antidote for modern-day stress.

Incorporating Movement Into Daily Life

One of the most common misconceptions about exercise is that it requires a gym membership or hours of free time. In reality, movement can be seamlessly integrated into daily routines. Simple habits, like taking the stairs instead of the elevator, parking farther away from entrances, or incorporating stretching breaks during work, can add up to significant health benefits. This section provides examples of how small, consistent changes can lead to a more active lifestyle without overwhelming commitments.

Finding Joy in Movement

Sustaining an exercise routine depends on finding activities that are enjoyable and personally rewarding. This section discusses how to explore different forms of movement, from dancing and swimming to hiking and team sports. For readers who find traditional workouts monotonous, activities like gardening, yoga, or even playing with pets can provide meaningful opportunities for physical activity. The focus is on discovering movement that feels less like a chore and more like a source of joy.

Structured Exercise for Different Fitness Levels

While incidental activity is beneficial, structured exercise plans can provide more targeted health benefits. This section introduces different types of exercise—cardiovascular, strength training, flexibility, and balance—and explains their unique contributions to overall health. Readers are guided on how to tailor workout plans to their fitness levels and goals. For beginners, this might mean starting with short, low-intensity sessions, while those with more experience can explore interval training or resistance exercises.

Overcoming Barriers to Exercise

For many, the biggest challenge to regular physical activity is overcoming barriers such as lack of time, motivation, or resources. This section addresses common obstacles and offers practical solutions. Readers learn strategies like breaking workouts into shorter sessions, finding accountability partners, and using bodyweight exercises that require no equipment. By addressing these challenges, the chapter empowers readers to view exercise as an achievable and sustainable practice.

The Importance of Rest and Recovery

Exercise is most effective when paired with adequate rest and recovery. This section emphasizes the role of rest days in preventing burnout and allowing the body to repair and strengthen. Stretching, foam rolling, and practices like yoga are discussed as ways to enhance flexibility and reduce muscle soreness. Recovery is framed as an integral part of any exercise routine, ensuring long-term sustainability, and preventing injury.

Movement Across Different Life Stages

The benefits of movement apply to all ages, but the approach to exercise should adapt to different life stages. For children, activities like play and sports build foundational fitness and coordination. In adulthood, exercise helps maintain strength and energy while mitigating health risks. For older adults, movement preserves mobility, balance, and independence. This section provides insights into tailoring exercise routines to suit the unique needs of each stage of life.

The Role of Technology in Encouraging Movement

Modern technology offers innovative ways to integrate and track physical activity. Fitness apps, wearable trackers, and online workout programs make it easier than ever to stay active. Readers learn how to use these tools to set goals, monitor progress, and stay motivated. Whether it's tracking steps with a smartwatch or joining a virtual exercise class, technology bridges the gap between intention and action.

Movement as a Lifelong Commitment

The chapter concludes by emphasizing that movement is a lifelong journey, not a short-term goal. Consistency, rather than intensity, is what yields lasting benefits. Readers are encouraged to approach exercise as a form of self-care and to celebrate every step toward a more active and healthier lifestyle. By viewing movement as medicine, they can transform their relationship with exercise and unlock its full potential to enhance their well-being.

This chapter leaves readers inspired and equipped to make physical activity a natural, rewarding part of their lives, paving the way for a healthier, more vibrant future.

Chapter 6: Mental Health and Emotional Resilience

Mental health is an integral part of overall well-being, yet it is often overlooked or stigmatized. Emotional resilience—the ability to adapt to life's challenges and recover from setbacks—is a skill that can be nurtured and strengthened over time. This chapter delves into the critical importance of mental health, offering practical strategies for managing stress, anxiety, and depression while fostering a deeper sense of emotional balance and resilience.

Understanding Mental Health and Its Impact

Mental health affects every aspect of our lives, from how we think and feel to how we interact with others and approach challenges. It is not merely the absence of illness but a state of emotional, psychological, and social well-being. This section explores the interconnectedness of mental and physical health, highlighting how chronic stress and unresolved emotional struggles can lead to physical ailments such as high blood pressure, digestive problems, and weakened immunity. Understanding the profound impact of mental health is the first step toward prioritizing and caring for it.

Managing Stress: Breaking the Cycle

Stress is a natural response to life's demands, but chronic stress can take a toll on the mind and body. This section explains the physiological effects of stress, such as elevated cortisol levels, and how they contribute to fatigue, irritability, and health issues. Strategies for managing stress are introduced, including time management, relaxation techniques, and setting boundaries. Readers are encouraged to identify their stress triggers and develop personalized coping mechanisms that help break the cycle of chronic stress.

Navigating Anxiety: Finding Calm in the Chaos

Anxiety, characterized by excessive worry or fear, is one of the most common mental health challenges. This section explores the signs of anxiety and how it differs from everyday stress. Techniques for reducing anxiety are introduced, such as deep breathing exercises, progressive muscle relaxation, and grounding techniques that bring focus to the present moment. Readers learn how to create safe spaces in their lives, both physically and emotionally, where they can retreat and recalibrate when feelings of anxiety arise.

Understanding and Addressing Depression

Depression, often referred to as the "silent illness," affects millions of people worldwide. This section discusses the symptoms of depression, such as persistent sadness, loss of interest in activities, and changes in appetite or sleep patterns. Practical strategies for addressing depression are explored, including establishing routines, engaging in physical activity, and finding small sources of joy. While these techniques can help, the section emphasizes the importance of seeking professional support when symptoms persist or worsen.

The Power of Mindfulness

Mindfulness—the practice of staying present and fully engaged in the moment—has gained recognition as a powerful tool for mental health. This section introduces readers to mindfulness practices, such as meditation, mindful breathing, and body scans. These techniques help individuals slow down racing thoughts, reduce stress, and gain clarity. Readers are encouraged to incorporate mindfulness into daily routines, whether through formal meditation sessions or simply savoring the moment during a walk or meal.

Journaling as a Therapeutic Tool

Writing down thoughts and emotions can be a powerful way to process and release mental burdens. This section explores the therapeutic benefits of journaling, from gaining insight into recurring patterns to setting intentions and goals. Readers are guided on how to start a journaling practice, whether by writing freely about their feelings, listing things they're grateful for, or documenting challenges and solutions. Journaling becomes a safe space for self-expression and reflection, fostering emotional resilience.

Building and Relying on Social Support

Human connection is fundamental to emotional resilience. This section emphasizes the importance of building and maintaining strong relationships with friends, family, and community. It explores how sharing challenges and seeking support can provide comfort and perspective during difficult times. Readers are encouraged to strengthen their social networks by reaching out to loved ones, participating in group activities, or seeking support groups that align with their experiences.

Recognizing When Professional Help Is Needed

While self-care strategies are valuable, there are times when professional mental health support is essential. This section discusses the signs that indicate a need for therapy or counseling, such as persistent feelings of hopelessness, difficulty functioning in daily life, or thoughts of self-harm. Readers are guided on how to find qualified mental health professionals, understand the different types of therapy available, and overcome the stigma often associated with seeking help.

Cultivating Emotional Resilience

Emotional resilience is the ability to bounce back from adversity and maintain a sense of balance in the face of challenges. This section explains how resilience is not an innate trait but a skill that can be developed through intentional practices. Strategies for building resilience include maintaining a positive outlook, learning from setbacks, and practicing self-compassion. Readers are encouraged to view challenges as opportunities for growth and to focus on their strengths rather than their limitations.

Creating a Mental Health Toolkit

A personalized mental health toolkit can provide resources for coping with difficult moments and maintaining emotional balance. This section encourages readers to identify practices, activities, and people that help them feel grounded and supported. From listening to music and engaging in creative outlets to practicing gratitude and setting achievable goals, the toolkit becomes a dynamic resource for managing mental health.

The Intersection of Mental and Physical Health

This section emphasizes the bidirectional relationship between mental and physical health. Engaging in regular physical activity, eating a balanced diet, and getting enough sleep are not only beneficial for the body but also have profound effects on mood and emotional well-being. Readers are reminded that caring for the mind and body together creates a holistic approach to health.

Moving Forward with Awareness and Care

The chapter concludes by encouraging readers to prioritize their mental health as an essential part of their overall well-being. By integrating mindfulness, self-reflection, and social connection into their lives, they can build the emotional resilience needed to navigate life's ups and downs. Readers are reminded that seeking support—whether from loved ones or professionals—is a sign of strength, not weakness. Mental health is a journey, and every small step toward self-care and awareness is a step toward a healthier, more balanced life.

Chapter 7: The Role of Regular Check-Ups

While self-care and daily health practices are essential, professional medical guidance plays a vital role in maintaining overall well-being. Regular check-ups are more than just routine appointments; they are proactive steps toward preventing illness, managing existing conditions, and ensuring long-term health. This chapter highlights the significance of these interactions with healthcare providers, offering insights on when to seek medical attention, how to make the most of appointments, and the importance of preventative screenings.

The Importance of Preventative Healthcare

Preventative healthcare focuses on identifying and addressing potential health issues before they become significant problems. Regular check-ups are the cornerstone of this approach, allowing doctors to detect early signs of illnesses such as hypertension, diabetes, and certain cancers. This section explains how preventative care extends beyond physical exams to include vaccinations, screenings, and lifestyle guidance. Readers are encouraged to view these visits not as reactive measures when they feel unwell but as essential tools for safeguarding their future health.

Knowing When to Seek Medical Attention

One of the most empowering aspects of self-care is knowing when professional medical attention is necessary. This section discusses the signs and symptoms that warrant a visit to the doctor, such as persistent fatigue, unexplained weight changes, or chronic pain. By recognizing these red flags, readers can avoid delaying care for potentially serious conditions. The section also emphasizes the importance of addressing minor concerns early, as they often reveal underlying issues that are easier to treat when caught early.

Establishing a Relationship with Your Healthcare Provider

A strong, trusting relationship with a healthcare provider is invaluable. This section explores how to select a primary care physician who aligns with your needs and values. Readers are guided on how to build rapport with their doctor, creating an open and collaborative dynamic. By fostering mutual respect and understanding, individuals can ensure that their medical care is personalized, comprehensive, and aligned with their health goals.

Communicating Effectively During Appointments

Maximizing the value of medical appointments requires effective communication. This section provides strategies for clearly expressing concerns, asking the right questions, and providing accurate information about symptoms and medical history. Readers are encouraged to prepare for visits by jotting down their questions and noting any changes in their health since their last appointment. Clear communication helps healthcare providers make informed decisions and ensures that patients leave with a clear understanding of their diagnosis and treatment plan.

The Role of Preventative Screenings

Preventative screenings are a crucial component of regular check-ups. From mammograms and colonoscopies to blood pressure and cholesterol tests, these screenings provide vital information about an individual's health. This section explains the purpose of various screenings, who should get them, and at what intervals. By demystifying the process, readers can approach these tests with confidence and understand their value in detecting and addressing health risks early.

The Emotional and Psychological Benefits of Regular Check-Ups

Beyond physical health, regular check-ups offer emotional reassurance. Knowing that a professional has evaluated your health and addressed potential concerns provides peace of mind. This section delves into the psychological benefits of preventative care, such as reduced anxiety about undiagnosed conditions. Readers are reminded that taking proactive steps for their health is an act of self-empowerment that contributes to overall well-being.

Tailoring Check-Ups to Life Stages

Health needs evolve over time, and regular check-ups should reflect these changes. This section examines how preventative care differs across various life stages. For children, check-ups focus on growth, development, and vaccinations. For adults, the emphasis shifts to screenings for chronic conditions, reproductive health, and lifestyle management. For older adults, check-ups address issues such as bone density, cognitive health, and mobility. By understanding the specific goals of care at each stage, readers can approach these visits with a sense of purpose and preparedness.

Overcoming Barriers to Regular Check-Ups

Despite their importance, many people neglect regular check-ups due to barriers such as time constraints, financial concerns, or fear of bad news. This section addresses these challenges head-on, offering practical solutions and encouraging readers to prioritize their health. Whether it's scheduling appointments well in advance, exploring insurance options, or reframing check-ups as opportunities for empowerment, this section helps readers navigate obstacles that might otherwise deter them.

The Role of Technology in Modern Healthcare

Advances in technology have transformed the healthcare landscape, making check-ups more accessible and efficient. This section explores how telemedicine, online appointment scheduling, and electronic health records enhance the patient experience. Readers are introduced to the benefits of virtual consultations, which allow for routine care and follow-ups from the comfort of home. Technology, when used effectively, makes preventative care more seamless and patient centered.

Building a Proactive Healthcare Plan

Regular check-ups are most effective when part of a broader proactive healthcare plan. This section encourages readers to take an active role in their medical care by tracking their appointments, following through on recommendations, and maintaining open communication with their provider. Readers are reminded that their health is a collaborative effort between themselves and their healthcare team.

Integrating Professional Guidance with Self-Care

Self-care and professional medical care are not mutually exclusive; they complement each other. This section discusses how regular check-ups can inform and enhance self-care practices. For instance, a doctor's recommendation for more physical activity can inspire a tailored exercise routine, while a discussion about diet can refine nutrition habits. By integrating the expertise of healthcare providers with personal health practices, individuals can achieve a more holistic approach to well-being.

Empowering Readers to Take Charge of Their Health

The chapter concludes with a call to action, encouraging readers to view regular check-ups as essential investments in their health and future. By understanding their role in preventative care, communicating effectively, and staying proactive, individuals can build a strong foundation for long-term well-being. Regular check-ups are not just medical appointments—they are opportunities to partner with professionals, gain valuable insights, and take confident steps toward a healthier life.

Chapter 8: Recognizing Red Flags

Understanding the signals your body sends is a crucial aspect of maintaining health. While many symptoms are mild and self-limiting, others could indicate serious underlying issues requiring immediate medical attention. This chapter focuses on helping readers distinguish between minor health concerns and red flags that should not be ignored. Recognizing these warning signs can save lives, prevent complications, and empower individuals to act swiftly when necessary.

The Importance of Listening to Your Body

The body communicates through symptoms, signaling when something isn't functioning properly. While occasional aches, fatigue, or discomfort are normal, persistent or unusual symptoms are often a sign of deeper issues. This section introduces the concept of tuning into your body's cues, encouraging readers to trust their instincts when something feels off. Early intervention is critical, as it often leads to better outcomes and less invasive treatments.

Recognizing Chest Pain and Cardiac Symptoms

Chest pain is one of the most alarming symptoms and for good reason. It can indicate a range of issues, from minor muscular strain to life-threatening conditions like a heart attack. This section explains how to differentiate between types of chest pain. For example, sharp, localized pain that worsens with movement might suggest a musculoskeletal issue, while crushing or pressure-like pain radiating to the arms, neck, or jaw is a red flag for a cardiac event. Readers are urged to seek immediate medical attention if they experience chest pain accompanied by shortness of breath, dizziness, or sweating.

Unexplained Weight Loss

Sudden, significant weight loss without changes in diet or exercise is another symptom that warrants concern. While minor fluctuations in weight are normal, losing more than 5% of your body weight in a short time can signal serious conditions such as cancer, hyperthyroidism, or chronic infections like tuberculosis. This section guides readers on how to track weight changes and when to consult a healthcare provider for further evaluation.

Persistent Fatigue and Weakness

Fatigue is a common complaint, often linked to lifestyle factors like poor sleep or overwork. However, when fatigue becomes persistent and is not alleviated by rest, it can indicate underlying conditions such as anemia, hypothyroidism, or even mental health issues like depression. This section explains how to differentiate between everyday tiredness and debilitating fatigue that requires medical attention. Readers learn to recognize accompanying symptoms like shortness of breath, palpitations, or difficulty concentrating as potential red flags.

Neurological Symptoms: Headaches, Dizziness, and Confusion

Neurological symptoms can be subtle but are sometimes indicative of serious conditions. Severe or sudden headaches, especially those accompanied by nausea, vision changes, or weakness on one side of the body, may signal a stroke or aneurysm. Persistent dizziness or balance issues could point to inner ear problems or neurological disorders. This section emphasizes the urgency of seeking medical care for these symptoms and highlights the importance of acting quickly in emergencies like suspected strokes, where time-sensitive treatments can prevent long-term damage.

Digestive Warning Signs

Digestive issues are common but can sometimes indicate severe underlying conditions. Symptoms such as persistent abdominal pain, unexplained vomiting, blood in the stool, or difficulty swallowing require immediate attention. This section explains how to distinguish between benign conditions like indigestion and more serious concerns like gastrointestinal bleeding, ulcers, or obstructions. Readers are encouraged to monitor these symptoms closely and seek care when they persist or worsen.

Breathing Difficulties

Shortness of breath can arise from physical exertion or anxiety, but when it occurs suddenly, worsens over time, or is accompanied by chest pain or wheezing, it may signal a serious condition like pneumonia, asthma, or a pulmonary embolism. This section educates readers on how to identify abnormal breathing patterns and when to call emergency services for respiratory distress.

Signs of Infections

Fever, chills, and localized swelling are common indicators of infection. While many infections resolve on their own or with antibiotics, some can escalate to sepsis, a life-threatening systemic response. This section guides readers on how to recognize warning signs of severe infections, such as a high fever, rapid heart rate, or confusion. Acting promptly in these cases can prevent complications and save lives.

Mental Health Red Flags

Mental health symptoms can be just as urgent as physical ones. Persistent feelings of hopelessness, withdrawal from loved ones, or thoughts of self-harm are signs that professional help is needed immediately. This section emphasizes the importance of addressing mental health concerns without delay and provides resources for seeking support.

When to Trust Your Instincts

Sometimes, symptoms may not fit neatly into a specific category but still feel concerning. This section encourages readers to trust their instincts and err on the side of caution. Even when symptoms seem vague, unexplained changes in how one feels or functions should not be ignored. Seeking a professional opinion can provide peace of mind and catch potential problems early.

Preparing for Medical Emergencies

Recognizing red flags is only part of the equation; knowing how to respond is equally important. This section provides practical advice on preparing for emergencies, such as keeping a list of medications and medical history readily available, knowing how to describe symptoms clearly, and understanding when to call emergency services versus visiting urgent care. Empowering readers with this knowledge ensures they are ready to act decisively in critical situations.

Proactive Awareness and Lifelong Vigilance

The chapter concludes by emphasizing that recognizing red flags is not about living in fear but about being proactive and attentive to the body's signals. By staying vigilant and acting promptly, readers can take control of their health and ensure that minor issues don't escalate into major concerns. This awareness, combined with regular check-ups and a commitment to self-care, forms the foundation of a long, healthy, and balanced life. Recognizing red flags is a skill that can save lives, turning knowledge into power and prevention into protection.

Chapter 9: The Power of Lifestyle Choices

Every day, we make choices that shape our long-term health and well-being. From the foods we eat to the habits we cultivate, these seemingly small decisions accumulate over time, significantly impacting our quality of life. This chapter delves into the profound influence of lifestyle choices on health, exploring how intentional, positive changes can lead to transformative results. By understanding and implementing these principles, readers can take control of their lives and build a foundation for long-term wellness.

The Ripple Effect of Daily Habits

Lifestyle choices are not isolated decisions but part of a larger ripple effect. One positive habit often leads to others, while negative choices can spiral into compounding health issues. For example, choosing to incorporate more whole foods into one's diet can lead to increased energy, which may inspire more physical activity. Conversely, sedentary behavior or poor dietary habits can increase the risk of obesity, heart disease, and mental health challenges. This section emphasizes how cumulative changes, whether positive or negative, influence long-term health outcomes.

Avoiding Smoking: A Lifesaving Choice

Smoking remains one of the leading preventable causes of illness and death worldwide. This section examines the far-reaching effects of tobacco use, from its role in respiratory and cardiovascular diseases to its links with various cancers. For those who smoke, quitting is one of the most impactful lifestyles changes they can make. Readers are guided on how to seek support, use cessation aids, and build a smoke-free environment. For non-smokers, avoiding exposure to secondhand smoke is equally critical, as its dangers are often underestimated.

Limiting Alcohol Intake

While moderate alcohol consumption may have social or cultural value, excessive drinking poses serious health risks, including liver disease, high blood pressure, and mental health disorders. This section explores how alcohol affects the body and mind, emphasizing the importance of moderation. Readers are encouraged to evaluate their drinking habits, set limits, and seek healthier ways to relax or socialize. For those struggling with dependency, resources and support systems are highlighted to facilitate recovery and sustainable change.

The Importance of Hobbies and Recreation

Engaging in hobbies and recreational activities is more than just a pastime—it is essential for mental and emotional well-being. This section explores how hobbies reduce stress, enhance creativity, and foster a sense of accomplishment. Whether it's gardening, painting, hiking, or playing a musical instrument, dedicating time to personal interests improves mood and resilience. Readers are encouraged to reconnect with activities that bring them joy and to prioritize leisure as a form of self-care.

Building Strong Relationships

The quality of our relationships has a profound effect on our health. Positive, supportive connections with family, friends, and community contribute to emotional stability, reduce stress, and even improve physical health outcomes. This section examines how loneliness and social isolation can lead to poor mental and physical health, while nurturing relationships can provide a buffer against life's challenges. Practical advice on strengthening existing bonds and forming new connections is offered, underscoring the value of meaningful human interactions.

The Role of Sleep in Lifestyle Choices

Sleep is often overlooked in discussions about lifestyle, yet it is a cornerstone of health. Poor sleep patterns can disrupt nearly every system in the body, leading to fatigue, weakened immunity, and increased risk of chronic diseases. This section highlights the importance of consistent, restorative sleep and provides strategies for improving sleep hygiene, such as establishing a regular bedtime routine, creating a comfortable sleep environment, and managing stress.

Nutrition and Its Daily Impact

What we eat fuels our bodies and minds, making dietary choices a pivotal aspect of lifestyle. This section explores how balanced, nutrient-rich meals support overall health and reduce the risk of chronic diseases. Simple tips for incorporating more fruits, vegetables, whole grains, and lean proteins into daily meals are provided, along with suggestions for reducing processed foods and added sugars. Readers are reminded that small, consistent changes, such as swapping sugary snacks for nuts or opting for water instead of soda, can lead to significant long-term benefits.

Physical Activity as a Daily Choice

Movement is medicine and integrating physical activity into daily routines is one of the most effective ways to improve health. This section examines the benefits of regular exercise, from enhanced cardiovascular health to improved mood and energy levels. Readers are encouraged to find activities they enjoy, whether it's walking, cycling, yoga, or dancing, and to view movement as an opportunity for self-care rather than a chore.

Stress Management Through Lifestyle

Chronic stress takes a toll on the body and mind, contributing to numerous health issues. This section explores how lifestyle choices can alleviate stress and build resilience. Techniques such as mindfulness, journaling, and spending time in nature are discussed as effective ways to reduce stress and enhance emotional well-being. Readers are encouraged to set boundaries, delegate tasks, and prioritize self-care to create a balanced, fulfilling life.

The Role of Gratitude and Mindset

A positive outlook can significantly influence lifestyle choices and overall health. This section examines how cultivating gratitude and practicing mindfulness can shift perspectives, making it easier to adopt and sustain healthy habits. Readers are guided on how to develop a gratitude practice, such as keeping a daily journal of things they appreciate, to foster a mindset that supports growth and well-being.

Cumulative Changes and Long-Term Benefits

The power of lifestyle choices lies in their cumulative effect. This section emphasizes that small, consistent actions—choosing water over soda, taking the stairs instead of the elevator, or spending ten minutes meditating—add up over time to create significant improvements in health and quality of life. Readers are encouraged to focus on progress rather than perfection and to celebrate every step toward positive change.

Living a Life of Intentional Choices

The chapter concludes by encouraging readers to approach their lives with intention. By making mindful, health-conscious decisions every day, they can shape a future that is vibrant, fulfilling, and resilient. Readers are reminded that while they cannot control every aspect of their health, the choices they make have the power to transform their lives, one small decision at a time.

Chapter 10: Advocating for Your Health

In a complex and often intimidating healthcare system, becoming your own advocate is essential. Navigating medical appointments, understanding diagnoses, and making informed decisions about treatments require confidence and knowledge. This chapter empowers readers to take an active role in their health care by teaching them how to communicate effectively with providers, seek clarity when needed, and make decisions that align with their values and goals.

Understanding the Importance of Health Advocacy

Health advocacy is about ensuring your voice is heard and your needs are met in the healthcare process. It involves being proactive, informed, and assertive while collaborating with medical professionals. This section explains why advocacy is crucial, particularly in systems where time with healthcare providers is limited, and the burden of understanding complex medical information often falls on the patient. Readers are encouraged to view themselves as equal partners in their care, capable of shaping their health journey through informed choices.

Preparing for Medical Appointments

A key aspect of health advocacy is preparing for medical appointments to make the most of the limited time with providers. This section guides readers on how to organize their thoughts, track symptoms, and bring relevant medical records to consultations. By arriving prepared, individuals can ensure that their concerns are addressed and that they leave with a clear understanding of their condition and next steps. Practical tips, such as keeping a health journal or using apps to log symptoms, are introduced to streamline this process.

Asking the Right Questions

Effective communication is the cornerstone of health advocacy. This section emphasizes the importance of asking thoughtful and specific questions during appointments. Readers are encouraged to inquire about the nature of their diagnosis, the purpose of prescribed treatments, potential side effects, and alternatives to suggested procedures. Open-ended questions, such as "What are the risks and benefits of this treatment?" or "Are there lifestyle changes I can make to improve my condition?" allow for more detailed and helpful responses. The section highlights the value of taking notes or bringing a trusted friend or family member to appointments for support.

Seeking Second Opinions

Sometimes, medical decisions can feel overwhelming, particularly when dealing with serious diagnoses or complex treatment plans. This section reassures readers that seeking a second opinion is not a sign of distrust but a responsible step in making informed decisions. It explains how second opinions can provide alternative perspectives, confirm diagnoses, or reveal additional treatment options. Readers learn how to approach this process respectfully, ensuring they maintain a positive relationship with their primary provider while exploring other expert insights.

Understanding Medical Bills and Insurance

Healthcare costs can be a significant source of confusion and stress. This section demystifies medical bills and insurance policies, helping readers understand terms like deductibles, co-pays, and out-of-pocket maximums. By becoming familiar with their coverage, readers can avoid unexpected expenses and make more informed decisions about where and how they receive care. The section also offers advice on how to dispute billing errors, negotiate costs, and seek financial assistance when necessary.

Advocating for Preventative Care

Preventative care is a critical yet often underutilized component of healthcare. This section encourages readers to advocate for regular screenings, vaccinations, and wellness visits, even when they feel healthy. By staying proactive, individuals can detect potential issues early and avoid more invasive and costly treatments later. Readers are reminded that advocacy extends beyond treating illness—it includes prioritizing measures that support long-term health and wellness.

Navigating Complex Healthcare Systems

Healthcare systems can be overwhelming, especially when navigating multiple specialists, facilities, or insurance requirements. This section provides strategies for managing these complexities, such as maintaining an organized file of medical records, test results, and insurance documents. Readers learn the value of keeping an open line of communication between different providers to ensure coordinated care. For those dealing with chronic or serious conditions, the role of patient advocates or case managers is discussed as a valuable resource.

Balancing Respect and Assertiveness

Advocating for your health requires a delicate balance between respecting medical professionals' expertise and asserting your own needs and preferences. This section explores how to express concerns, request additional information, or decline certain treatments without damaging the doctor-patient relationship. Readers are encouraged to trust their instincts while remaining open to guidance, creating a partnership that prioritizes their best interests.

The Role of Technology in Health Advocacy

Advances in technology have made it easier for individuals to access and manage their health information. This section explores how patient portals, telemedicine, and health apps empower readers to take control of their care. For instance, patient portals allow individuals to review test results, communicate with providers, and schedule appointments online, reducing the barriers to active participation. Telemedicine offers convenience and accessibility, particularly for follow-ups or consultations with specialists in different locations.

Recognizing Your Rights as a Patient

Understanding patient rights is a fundamental aspect of health advocacy. This section informs readers about their rights to privacy, informed consent, and access to medical records. It explains how these rights protect individuals and empower them to make decisions aligned with their values. Readers are encouraged to speak up if they feel their rights are being violated and to seek support from patient advocacy groups when necessary.

Advocating for Loved Ones

Health advocacy often extends beyond oneself, particularly when caring for children, elderly parents, or loved ones with complex medical needs. This section provides guidance on how to advocate effectively for others, ensuring they receive appropriate care and that their preferences are respected. Readers learn how to communicate with providers on behalf of loved ones, coordinate care, and support decision-making in a compassionate and respectful manner.

Embracing Health Advocacy as a Lifelong Skill

The chapter concludes by emphasizing that health advocacy is a lifelong skill that evolves with changing needs and circumstances. Readers are encouraged to view advocacy not as a one-time action but as an ongoing commitment to their well-being. By taking an active role in their healthcare, they can build stronger partnerships with providers, make informed decisions, and ensure that their health journey reflects their unique goals and priorities. Advocacy is not just about navigating the healthcare system—it is about reclaiming agency and confidence in managing one's own health.

Chapter 11: Empowering Your Family to Be Their Own Physicians

Health and wellness are not just individual pursuits—they are deeply rooted in the habits, values, and practices shared within a family. This chapter extends the book's principles to family health, offering readers practical strategies to foster a culture of wellness at home. By empowering each family member to understand and prioritize their health, families can collectively achieve long-term well-being and resilience.

The Family as a Unit of Wellness

Families are the foundation of lifelong habits and creating a culture of health at home starts with understanding that wellness is a shared responsibility. This section introduces the concept of the family as a unit of wellness, where each member plays a role in fostering a supportive environment. When families work together to prioritize health, they not only improve individual outcomes but also strengthen their emotional connections and collective resilience.

Building Awareness Across Generations

Health education often focuses on adults, but empowering family members of all ages—from children to grandparents—is essential for comprehensive wellness. This section explores how to teach children the basics of self-care, such as understanding the importance of hygiene, eating nutritious meals, and recognizing when they're unwell. At the same time, it emphasizes the importance of involving older generations in health discussions, ensuring that everyone feels valued and informed about their health decisions.

Meal Planning for the Whole Family

Nutrition is a cornerstone of family health, and meal planning provides an opportunity to involve everyone in making healthier choices. This section discusses how families can work together to create balanced, nutrient-rich meals that cater to diverse preferences and dietary needs. Readers learn practical tips for grocery shopping, cooking together, and incorporating seasonal, whole foods into their diets. When meal planning becomes a collaborative activity, it fosters accountability and reinforces the importance of good nutrition for everyone.

Encouraging Family Exercise

Physical activity is vital for maintaining health and incorporating exercise into family routines can make it enjoyable and sustainable. This section explores various ways to engage the whole family in physical activity, from weekend hikes and bike rides to home workout sessions and dance nights. It highlights the importance of modeling active behavior for children and creating a positive association with exercise. By turning movement into a shared experience, families build habits that benefit everyone's physical and mental health.

Creating a Healthy Home Environment

A family's environment plays a significant role in shaping health behaviors. This section discusses how to create a home that supports wellness, including reducing clutter, ensuring access to healthy foods, and setting aside screen-free zones for relaxation and connection. Readers learn how to make small but impactful changes, such as incorporating indoor plants to improve air quality or establishing a quiet space for meditation or reading. These changes create a nurturing atmosphere that encourages health-conscious choices.

Open Communication About Health

Open communication is the foundation of empowering family members to take charge of their health. This section emphasizes the importance of discussing health openly and without stigma, encouraging conversations about physical symptoms, emotional well-being, and health goals. When families normalize these discussions, they reduce barriers to seeking help and make it easier for everyone to feel supported. Readers are guided on how to foster a judgment-free environment where all members feel comfortable sharing their concerns.

Teaching the Importance of Preventative Care

Preventative care is a family effort, and this section explores how to involve all members in regular check-ups, vaccinations, and screenings. By teaching children, the importance of visiting the doctor for wellness check-ups rather than only when they're sick, parents can instill a proactive approach to health. Similarly, adults can model this behavior by prioritizing their own preventative care, showing the value of addressing potential health issues before they arise.

Encouraging Emotional and Mental Well-Being

Family health goes beyond the physical—it includes emotional and mental well-being. This section addresses how families can support one another through stress, anxiety, and life's challenges. Techniques like practicing mindfulness together, engaging in group relaxation activities, and openly discussing emotions are explored as ways to strengthen emotional resilience. Readers learn how to recognize signs of mental distress in family members and encourage seeking professional help when needed.

Managing Chronic Conditions as a Family

Chronic conditions often affect more than just the individual—they impact the entire family. This section discusses how families can support members with chronic illnesses, such as diabetes, asthma, or arthritis, by creating a unified approach to care. Whether it's adjusting meal plans, scheduling medication reminders, or participating in low-impact exercises, the collective effort helps alleviate the burden on the individual while reinforcing family bonds.

Fostering Independence in Health

While families are a source of support, it is equally important to encourage individual responsibility for health. This section explores how to teach children, teenagers, and even aging parents to take an active role in their well-being. By empowering each member to make informed decisions—such as reading food labels, setting fitness goals, or managing medications—families cultivate independence and self-reliance in health care.

Celebrating Progress Together

Celebrating milestones and progress as a family reinforces positive behaviors and motivates everyone to stay committed to their health goals. This section suggests ways to acknowledge achievements, such as completing a fitness challenge, cooking healthier meals for a month, or overcoming a health issue. By celebrating together, families create a sense of accomplishment and inspire each other to continue striving for wellness.

Creating a Legacy of Wellness

The chapter concludes by highlighting the long-term impact of fostering a culture of health within families. When families prioritize wellness, they create a legacy that extends across generations, teaching children and grandchildren the value of self-care and mutual support. Readers are reminded that empowering their family to be their own physicians is not just about immediate benefits—it's about building a healthier, happier future for everyone. Through collaboration, communication, and shared commitment, families can thrive together, equipped to face life's challenges with strength and resilience.

Conclusion: A Call to Take Charge of Your Health

As the journey through this book ends, the most important takeaway is clear: every individual possesses the power to take charge of their health. This is not merely about managing symptoms or responding to illness but about proactively building a foundation for lifelong well-being. By becoming the primary care physician for themselves, readers can transform their lives, making choices that empower them to live healthier, happier, and more fulfilling lives.

The Power of Personal Agency

The central message of this book has been the importance of personal agency in health. Readers have learned how to listen to their bodies, identify red flags, and use the tools and knowledge at their disposal to make informed decisions. The power to improve health does not reside solely in doctors' offices or medical systems—it lies within each person's ability to take small, consistent steps toward better living. Whether it's adjusting nutrition, prioritizing exercise, or managing stress, the cumulative effect of these actions is profound.

A Reflection on Key Lessons

Throughout the book, readers have explored the pillars of preventative care, the role of nutrition and exercise, the importance of regular check-ups, and the need to advocate for their health. They have been equipped with strategies to recognize early warning signs, foster emotional resilience, and empower their families to adopt a culture of wellness. These lessons are interconnected, forming a comprehensive approach to self-care that places the individual at the center of their health journey.

Case studies from real-life experiences illustrate these principles in action. For instance, one individual recognized early symptoms of prediabetes and used the guidance in this book to make dietary and lifestyle changes, ultimately reversing the condition without medication. Another case study highlights a family that implemented regular wellness practices, from meal planning to group exercise, creating a healthier environment for every member. These stories serve as reminders that change is possible and within reach.

Tools for Continued Growth

To help readers implement what they have learned, practical worksheets and tools are included as resources for ongoing self-care. These worksheets guide readers in tracking their health metrics, setting achievable goals, and reflecting on their progress. For example, a "Daily Health Tracker" allows readers to log meals, exercise, hydration, and emotional well-being, while a "Symptom Journal" helps identify patterns and triggers that may require attention. These tools make it easier to stay engaged and committed to their health journey.

For those seeking deeper insights, additional chapters can be included to address specific topics such as managing chronic illnesses, navigating menopause or andropause, and fostering health equity in diverse communities. By expanding the scope of the book, readers with unique needs can find tailored guidance that resonates with their experiences.

The Ripple Effect of Health Ownership

Taking charge of personal health has a ripple effect, benefiting not only the individual but also their families, workplaces, and communities. When one person adopts healthier habits, it often inspires those around them to do the same. This creates a collective shift toward wellness that extends far beyond the individual, fostering a culture where health is prioritized and celebrated. Readers are reminded that by becoming role models for self-care, they contribute to a larger movement of proactive, informed health management.

Embracing Imperfection and Growth

While this book provides a roadmap to better health, it acknowledges that the journey is not always linear. Life's demands, setbacks, and unexpected challenges can sometimes disrupt even the best-laid plans. Readers are encouraged to embrace imperfection and view each day as an opportunity to start anew. Growth is not about perfection but about persistence, and every small step matters.

A Vision for the Future

The ultimate vision of this book is a world where individuals are empowered to be the primary stewards of their health. In this world, people listen to their bodies, advocate for their needs, and work collaboratively with healthcare providers to achieve optimal well-being. This vision is not aspirational—it is achievable, and it begins with the choices each person makes today.

Closing Words

As readers close this book, they are invited to take the first step toward becoming the primary care physician for themselves. Whether it's scheduling a long-overdue check-up, incorporating more whole foods into their diet, or starting a mindfulness practice, every action counts. The journey to better health is not a sprint but a lifelong adventure, and each reader has the tools, knowledge, and power to navigate it with confidence.

By embracing this call to action, readers not only improve their physical and mental well-being but also unlock the potential for a richer, more fulfilling life. This is more than just self-care—it is self-empowerment, and it is the key to living well. With this mindset, readers can move forward, equipped to thrive, and inspire others to do the same.

The role of your PCP

The primary role of a Primary Care Physician (PCP) is to be the main point of contact for a patient's healthcare needs. PCPs provide comprehensive, ongoing, and personalized care, focusing on prevention, diagnosis, treatment, and coordination of care. Key responsibilities include:

Preventive Care:

Conducting routine check-ups, screenings, and vaccinations to prevent illnesses and detect health issues early.

Diagnosis and Treatment:

Evaluating symptoms, diagnosing conditions, and providing treatment for a wide range of acute and chronic illnesses.

Health Education:

Guiding patients on lifestyle choices, such as diet, exercise, stress management, and other factors to promote wellness.

Care Coordination:

Acting as a liaison between the patient and specialists or other healthcare providers, ensuring coordinated and holistic care.

Managing Chronic Conditions:

Monitoring and managing long-term conditions like diabetes, hypertension, or asthma, and adjusting treatments as necessary.

Building a Long-Term Relationship:

Developing a deep understanding of a patient's health history, preferences, and needs to provide personalized and effective care.

A PCP plays a pivotal role in advocating for a patient's overall health, emphasizing a proactive approach to wellness rather than reactive treatment.

Where there is no doctor…

In the absence of a Primary Care Physician (PCP), taking proactive responsibility for your own health becomes essential. This involves understanding and monitoring your body, making informed decisions, and seeking professional assistance when necessary. Here's how to embody the role of your own PCP:

Prevention: Be Proactive, Not Reactive

Learn About Your Body: Understand your normal body functions (e.g., weight, sleep patterns, energy levels, appetite, digestion).

Healthy Lifestyle Choices:

Nutrition: Eat a balanced diet rich in fruits, vegetables, lean proteins, and whole grains.

Exercise: Stay active with regular physical activity suited to your abilities.

Sleep Hygiene: Prioritize quality sleep (7-9 hours for most adults).

Stress Management: Practice mindfulness, yoga, or other relaxation techniques.

Avoid Risk Factors: Minimize alcohol, avoid smoking, and limit exposure to environmental toxins.

Monitor Your Health

Track Your Symptoms: Keep a journal of symptoms, changes in your body, or unusual feelings.

Self-Screening: Regularly check for lumps, skin changes, or any abnormalities.

Measure Key Indicators: If accessible, monitor blood pressure, blood sugar, weight, and temperature.

Educate Yourself

Health Literacy: Learn about common illnesses, their symptoms, and preventive measures.

Use Reliable Sources: Refer to reputable health websites (e.g., WHO, CDC) or books to understand health topics.

Act as Your Health Advocate

Ask Questions: Seek to understand what your body is telling you when you feel unwell.

Challenge Assumptions: Explore potential causes of symptoms rather than immediately dismissing them.

Stay Informed: Keep up to date with health guidelines, vaccination schedules, and community health updates.

Seek Alternatives to a PCP

Community Resources: Leverage nurses, pharmacists, or community health workers for advice.

Telemedicine: Use online health consultations if available.

Peer Support Groups: Connect with others managing similar health concerns for shared learning.

Build a Personal Health Plan

Set Goals: Create achievable health objectives, such as improving diet or increasing exercise.

Create Checklists: Include routines for dental care, hygiene, and regular self-assessments.

Maintain Records: Keep copies of past health records, vaccination history, and medical test results.

Recognize When to Seek Help

Emergencies: Know when to seek urgent care for symptoms like severe pain, chest tightness, or difficulty breathing.

Persistent Issues: For ongoing or worsening symptoms, find access to a healthcare professional or clinic.

Listen to Your Body

Trust your instincts. You are the expert on how you feel day-to-day and recognizing changes early can prevent complications.

By integrating these practices into your routine, you effectively act as your own PCP, taking charge of your health while being prepared to collaborate with professionals if needed. This approach emphasizes the power of self-awareness and informed decision-making in maintaining wellness.

I am the PCP of my body; any other care provider is a secondary care provider (SCP)

The statement, *"I am the PCP of my body; any other care provider is a secondary care provider (SCP),"* reflects a profound perspective on personal health responsibility. It emphasizes self-awareness and active engagement in one's well-being, where you take the lead in understanding and maintaining your health. Here's an analysis of this idea:

The Core Truth: You Are Your Body's Best Advocate

Self-Knowledge is Primary:

No one knows your body better than you. You feel its subtle changes, rhythms, and signals long before they can be measured or diagnosed by others.

Primary Source of Information:

Healthcare providers rely heavily on the information you provide—symptoms, lifestyle choices, and medical history. Your accurate reporting is foundational to effective care.

Empowerment Through Awareness:

By taking charge, you empower yourself to make informed decisions about your health and treatment, avoiding unnecessary reliance on others.

Shifting the Paradigm: From Passive to Active Participation

In traditional models, PCPs lead health management, and patients follow instructions. The statement redefines this by placing **you** in the driver's seat, with other care providers playing supportive or consultative roles.

This approach requires:

Proactive Engagement: Monitoring your health and seeking preventive care.

Health Literacy: Understanding basic medical concepts, risk factors, and symptoms.

Informed Decision-Making: Weighing the benefits and risks of treatments or lifestyle changes.

Benefits of Being Your Own PCP

Personalized Care:

Your decisions are based on your unique needs and preferences rather than generalized medical protocols.

Cost Efficiency:

Preventive self-care can reduce unnecessary medical visits and interventions.

Improved Communication:

Understanding your health better allows for more effective collaboration with SCPs.

Resilience in Low-Resource Settings:

In areas with limited healthcare access, this mindset fosters independence and problem-solving.

The Role of Secondary Care Providers (SCPs)

While you are the "primary," SCPs bring **expertise**, **tools**, and **interventions** that complement your self-care:

Diagnosis and Treatment: For conditions beyond self-management.

Advanced Procedures: Surgery, specialized therapies, or diagnostic imaging.

Knowledge Gaps: Addressing areas where your understanding may fall short.

SCPs should be seen as **partners**, not leaders, in your health journey.

The Limitations of the Approach

While this philosophy empowers self-reliance, it's important to acknowledge its boundaries:

Lack of Expertise: You may not have the training to identify complex health issues.

Bias in Self-Assessment: Overconfidence in self-diagnosis can delay professional intervention.

Access to Resources: Advanced medical tools and treatments often require SCPs.

A balanced approach respects the complementary roles of self-care and professional care.

A Holistic Health Philosophy

Claiming the role of your body's PCP is a bold and empowering declaration of ownership over your well-being. It underscores the need for self-awareness, education, and responsibility. However, recognizing the value of SCPs ensures that your health strategy remains comprehensive and collaborative. Together, these roles—primary and secondary—create a robust framework for achieving and maintaining optimal health.

Your critique of the U.S. healthcare system reflects frustrations that many individuals share, particularly regarding its structure, accessibility, and financial motivations. Let's break this down for a balanced discussion:

Chapter 12: The Reality of Healthcare in the U.S.

Profit-Driven System:

The U.S. healthcare system operates largely as a for-profit model. Private insurance companies, pharmaceutical companies, and hospitals often prioritize revenue generation, which can overshadow patient-centered care.

Chronic conditions can indeed become revenue streams for the system, with ongoing treatments, prescriptions, and specialist visits encouraged instead of exploring preventive or holistic solutions.

Long Wait Times and Accessibility:

Emergency departments often experience overcrowding due to a combination of understaffing, high patient loads, and a lack of preventive care access.

Delays in accessing a PCP or specialist, particularly for non-urgent issues, are another glaring problem, exacerbated by administrative inefficiencies and a shortage of primary care physicians.

Insurance Challenges

Coverage Inequalities:

Insurance determines the quality of care many patients receive. Those with "good" coverage often receive more attention, but this doesn't always equate to better health outcomes—it may lead to unnecessary treatments or tests.

High Costs:

Even with insurance, patients often face high deductibles, co-pays, or surprise billing, leaving many underinsured or avoiding care altogether.

Medical Bankruptcy:

The U.S. is one of the few developed nations where medical expenses are a leading cause of bankruptcy, highlighting systemic flaws.

Preventive Care Neglected

Reactive vs. Proactive:

The system often focuses on treating illness rather than preventing it. Regular checkups, education on lifestyle changes, and early intervention are less emphasized because they don't generate immediate profits.

Chronic Condition Management:

Many patients are prescribed medications to "manage" symptoms rather than addressing root causes through diet, exercise, and other holistic approaches.

The Role of the Emergency Room

Overburdened ERs:

Emergency rooms in the U.S. often function as safety nets for uninsured or underinsured individuals who can't access primary care, leading to long wait times and resource strain.

Triage System:

The priority in emergency rooms is based on severity, meaning less critical patients may wait hours while more urgent cases are attended to.

Comparing with Other Countries

Universal Healthcare Models:

Many Western countries (e.g., Canada, the U.K., Germany) have universal healthcare systems where patients don't face the same financial barriers or insurance-driven care. These systems emphasize access and affordability over profit.

Medical Tourism:

Seeking care abroad can indeed be more affordable and effective for certain treatments. Countries like India, Thailand, or Mexico offers high-quality care at a fraction of U.S. costs.

Your Perspective: Self-Advocacy

Given your observations, your advice about being your own PCP gains even more relevance. Being proactive in managing your health can reduce reliance on a system that may prioritize profit over patient outcomes.

Educating oneself about treatment options, questioning recommendations, and considering second opinions can empower patients in navigating this complex system.

Hope for Change

Push for Reform:

There are ongoing discussions about healthcare reform in the U.S., with advocates pushing for systems like Medicare for All or expanded Affordable Care Act provisions.

Emphasis on Transparency:

Greater transparency in pricing, outcomes, and incentives could help align the system more closely with patient-centered care.

Your critique highlights critical shortcomings of the U.S. healthcare system, particularly its profit-driven nature, accessibility challenges, and systemic inefficiencies. While some healthcare providers prioritize patient care, the system itself often incentivizes financial gain over holistic well-being. Until meaningful reform occurs, individuals must remain vigilant, informed, and proactive about their health to navigate these challenges effectively.

USA Healthcare is a Political Commodity for Presidential Elections

Your observation that healthcare in the United States has become a political commodity is a critical and insightful point. Indeed, healthcare often dominates political campaigns, with promises of reform, cost reduction, and expanded access being central themes. However, as you suggest, there's often a gap between campaign rhetoric and actionable reform once candidates take office. Here's a deeper dive into this issue:

Healthcare as a Political Tool

Campaign Promises:

Politicians frequently use healthcare as a platform to connect with voters, capitalizing on widespread dissatisfaction with the system. Promises to lower costs, expand access, or introduce universal healthcare resonate strongly with the electorate.

Partisan Divide:

Healthcare policy in the U.S. is deeply polarized. Democrats often push for expanded public options like Medicare for All, while Republicans lean toward market-driven solutions and reducing government intervention. This divide often results in gridlock and little meaningful progress.

Exploitation of the System

Lobbying Influence:

After being elected, many politicians become enmeshed in a system heavily influenced by powerful healthcare lobbies, including insurance companies, pharmaceutical giants, and hospital corporations. These entities fund campaigns and exert pressure to maintain the status quo.

Profit Over Patients:

The for-profit nature of the U.S. healthcare system aligns well with political inaction, as significant reform could disrupt lucrative revenue streams for these industries.

Citizen Exploitation

Rising Costs:

Despite campaign promises, healthcare costs (insurance premiums, deductibles, prescription drugs) continue to rise, burdening average citizens and driving some into financial ruin.

Access Inequities:

Many Americans remain uninsured or underinsured, unable to afford necessary care despite living in one of the wealthiest nations in the world.

False Expectations:

Voters place trust in politicians who promise sweeping reforms but often receive piecemeal changes or policies that exacerbate systemic problems.

Lack of Accountability

Short-Term Gains:

Politicians may propose temporary fixes or highlight minor successes to appease constituents while avoiding long-term systemic changes that require substantial effort and political risk.

Manipulating Voter Sentiment:

By focusing on emotional appeals—such as stories of families struggling with medical bills—politicians gain voter support but fail to deliver comprehensive solutions.

Systemic Entrapment

Reinforcing the Status Quo:

Politicians who enter the system with genuine intentions may find themselves limited by institutional barriers, lobbying influence, and the political cost of challenging entrenched interests.

Healthcare as a Commodity:

The U.S. treats healthcare not as a human right but as a commodity, where access is often tied to employment, income, and geography. This commodification aligns with broader capitalist principles but leaves many Americans underserved.

The Need for Citizen Action

Demanding Accountability:

Citizens must hold politicians accountable for unfulfilled promises, pressing them for transparency and measurable outcomes.

Advocating for Reform:

Grassroots movements and advocacy for policies like universal healthcare, expanded Medicare, or increased transparency can drive the political agenda.

Educating Voters:

Raising awareness about the complexities of healthcare policy and the influence of corporate interests can empower voters to make informed choices.

The Global Contrast

Many developed nations treat healthcare as a basic right, providing universal coverage and focusing on patient outcomes rather than profit. This contrast highlights the unique challenges of the U.S. system and the role of political will in achieving reform.

Your critique underscores a fundamental issue: healthcare in the U.S. is more than just a service—it's a political pawn. Until the system prioritizes patient well-being over profits and political gains, citizens will continue to bear the burden. Meaningful change requires not only political courage but also a collective demand for accountability and fairness from voters and advocacy groups.